Rest... You Win

Rest...

You Win

"Come to me, all you who labor and are heavy laden and I will give you rest."

Matthew 11:8 NKJV

Suzanne Leigh

Rest…You Win

Copyright © 2021 by Suzanne Leigh

ISBN 13: 979-853-228-643-6
Independently Published
Suzanne Leigh
www.suzanneleigh.me

Unless otherwise noted, scripture quotations are taken from the New King James Version (NKJV).

Suzanne Leigh

Bringing Hope, Healing and Encouragment

Printed in the United States

This book is dedicated to my Mom

Mom, I was so blessed to have spent the past four years making memories with you. Life is short; forgive and love, these are the two most important things we can do in life, aside from inviting Christ into our hearts.
R.I.P. Mom

Dear Reader

In December of 2018, I released my first published work, Resilient 7 Stages of Growing in Faith. One month later, in 2019, I began my studies at Southeastern University in Lakeland, Florida. That summer, I sensed the Lord leading me to my next writing assignment. The word I received was REST. With 2020, toilet paper shortages, and much uncertainty, I not only completed most of the book, but I also completed my studies at Southeastern and graduated with a degree in Organizational Leadership in December 2020. Who knew? God knew what I needed. I learned a lot about myself during my studies, and I believe it reflects in my new book. God doesn't reveal every step beforehand; He waits until we've completed the first assignment before He reveals the next step.

To God be the Glory!

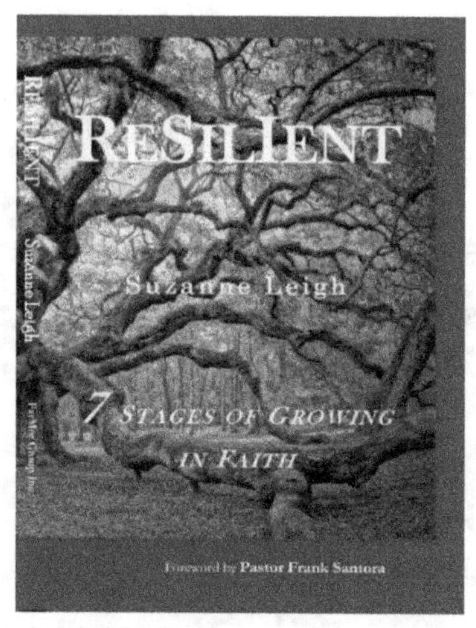

Scan the QR code to go directly to Amazon for the purchase of all books.

Rest…You Win Workbook available for download Aug. 2021 @ www.suzanneleigh.org

To contact or keep up with current and future writing and speaking engagements, please visit www.suzanneleigh.org

Table of Contents

Acknowledgments

I want to thank Toni for her creative digital edits and web design. I would also like to thank Suzette from FarMor Publishing for helping me get the words right, and a shout out to Roslyn Clark for advising me through the art of presentation.

I REST

I rest from worry; I rest from hurry, I rest from strife, I rest.

I rest from the offense; I rest from anger; I rest from confusion, I rest.

I rest in Your grace; I rest in Your peace, I rest in Your love, I rest.

I rest in Your faithfulness to uphold me in your righteous right hand, I rest.

I rest in the plans You have for me; I rest.

I stop trying to control how everything is going to work out; I rest.

I rest in knowing it's all working out for good. I keep my heart centered on You. I rest.

I rest in the finished work of the cross.

I rest in knowing I belong to the Father through Christ by the Spirit.

I rest in Your goodness to watch over me, care for me, lead me, and direct me.

I rest in my ability to hear You. I get quite long enough to listen to your direction for each day. I rest (in You God).

I rest from a restless soul. And as I tune into You, my soul rests.

II

III

Introduction

What do you see when you hear the word "rest?" Maybe you visualize taking a nap or the restful sounds and smells of the ocean, a massage, or some other relaxing cathartic. Rest is defined; by Webster's Dictionary as: to cease from work or movement to relax, refresh oneself, or recover strength. Synonyms include relax, take a load off, chillax, catch some z's, let up, slow down, take a break, unwind, recharge batteries, be at leisure, take it easy, kick your feet up, go to bed, take a nap, sleep, or take a breather.[1]

REST…You Win will discuss the natural form of rest and how the mental, emotional, and physical body are affected by both adequate and inadequate rest. Furthermore, we will consider the biblical intention of rest, according to the Old and New Testament, including the Sabbath Rest for man, His creation, and what it means to enter the rest of God. In the busyness of life, many are stuck in a rut of continual momentum, which includes work, school, home, provision for our families, upkeep of our homes, etc. This cycle of life, when added to the financial pressures of making ends meet, and the continual flow of information that bombards our minds, rest becomes a necessity.

Many people live on fumes, lacking the essential sleep requirements needed to rejuvenate the body. Just as food and water are sustainers of life, so is obtaining adequate amounts of rest.

Stress often causes aches and pains in the body, including fatigue, headaches, and upset stomach. It affects our moods, causing anxiety, depression, irritability, frustration, and anger. Stress from lack of rest can lead to outbursts of anger, overeating, alcohol, or drugs, and even withdrawal.[2] It is something to be managed, not something to be ignored. Poor nutrition, lack of sleep, and exercise are all culprits to many diseases people face. Often, we have been prescribed medicines for aliments when what we've failed to implement is exercise, nutrition, and proper rest. God created the earth with everything man needed to sustain a healthy existence, and rest is a part of the equation.

VI

1
REST FOR THE BODY

"In vain you rise early and stay up late, toiling for food to eat-- for He grants sleep to those He loves" **(Psalm 127:2, NIV)**.

Effects from Lack of Sleep

Proverbs 3:24,

> "When you lie down, you will not be afraid; when you lie down, your sleep will be sweet" (NIV).

What happens to the mind when we do not get adequate rest? According to the American Psychological Association (2018),[3] lack of sleep costs billions of dollars every year. The APA cites that 100,000 crashes per year are caused by persons falling asleep at the wheel, and 4% of those lead to death.

The Department of Transportation (DOT)[4] assigns a number to (registered) commercial vehicles, and it clocks truck drivers for their hours on the road. They are mandated to stop often for rest and sleep breaks. Driving in a state of lethargy is a violation of DOT regulations (with the same consequences, both mentally and physically, as driving under the influence of alcohol). If truck drivers do not comply with DOT regulations, they can be fined, or temporarily lose their operating privileges.[2]

Once, while driving to Atlanta in the middle of the night at the age of 19, I stopped to visit a friend in Gainesville, Florida. My plan was to leave earlier that evening. However, I left after 11 p.m. A couple of hours later, lethargy set in, but I pushed myself to keep driving. Somewhere in the mix, three semitrucks decided to play games, sandwiching me: one in front; one behind; and one on the left for 13 seemingly endless miles. As soon as the first exit presented itself, I escaped the trio to find a motel. The stress from staying awake was not easy. I thought it would never end, but when it did, I was relieved.

Sleeplessness and the Body

Ecclesiastes 2:23,

> "Because all his days his task is painful
> and grievous; even at night his mind
> does not rest. This too is vanity" (NASB).

Not only does lack of sleep contribute to highway accidents, but it also interferes with brain function and a person's ability to focus, reason, absorb, and recall information. Without adequate sleep, the body is unable to function optimally. Like a car that needs to be refueled, our bodies are created to be replenished regularly.

Lack of sleep on a consistent basis, less than 7-8 hours per night (more for youth and children), affects our brain and its ability to concentrate and problem solve. It also affects cognitive decisions and causes poor focus, and heightened agitation, slowed reflexes, decrease hormone regulation, increased glucose levels, and even obesity.[4] In fact, studies show that lack of sleep increases cortisol levels. You may be wondering, what is *cortisol*? Cortisol is better known as the "stress hormone"[5] that is initiated by the *fight or flight response.*

In normal everyday doses, cortisol has its benefits; "increase energy and focus."[5] However, in large amounts, over extended periods, cortisol causes "fatigue, irritability, headaches, gastric problems, anxiety, depression, weight gain, increased blood pressure, low libido, difficulty recovering from exercise, and poor sleep and even skin problems."[5]

Cortisol makes the heart work harder, increasing a person's risk for high cholesterol, heart attack, and stroke. Furthermore, sleep deprivation suppresses immune function, increasing risks for infection (colds, viruses, and other invaders). Lack of sleep also decreases the liver's ability to detox, thus affecting metabolism, of which the liver is responsible.[5] In addition, lack of sleep affects testosterone, thus decreasing a man's energy levels and strength, causing fatigue, increased insomnia, and even infertility. These are just a few factors from lack of sleep.[5]

Other culprits to insomnia are medications and coping mechanisms to stress, nicotine, alcohol, illegal drugs, caffeine, sugar, and comfort foods. Sometimes, making simple life adjustments can make all the difference, but first one must be aware of what habits are contributing to the problem. For example, eating chocolate or caffeine late in the afternoon can affect sleep.[3]

Recommendations

Although naps are rejuvenating (and can help to clear the mind and enable one to focus better on tasks), if taken too late in the day or too long, it causes sleeplessness. Have you had this problem? Limiting the time and duration of naps may help. According to an article on WebMD, to promote restful sleep, doctors recommend developing a regular routine for waking and sleep, avoiding caffeine, nicotine, alcohol, and certain foods prior to bedtime; and abstaining from watching TV, reading, and eating in bed.[7] Therefore, what we ingest into our bodies and minds does matter.

Financial Unrest

"A big part of financial freedom is having your heart and mind free from worry about what-ifs of life."[8]

Have you ever asked God for something, then became impatient waiting for it? Does it align with God's will, His word? Often, we are not even prepared to receive things we have asked God for. For example, if you want a million dollars, are you mature enough to handle that kind of money? Just because you do not have the things you've asked for, does not mean God is saying "No!" He may be preparing you to handle all you have asked for, and that takes time. And so, there is an opportune moment depending on whether you have done the groundwork. The Bible gives instruction in righteous living, and how to handle finances. When we handle our funds properly, there is peace, there is rest. However, many are anxious about their finances; not enough, always needing more?

Do you find yourself worried about finances?

The lack of savings is a high-stress factor. I remember a time when I was on an extremely limited budget. I had to learn how to live on little and get by. No credit cards to rely on; no savings; no longer qualified for food stamps; and I did not make enough to afford the extras. But God; He always supplied.

With a limited budget for food, we relied on less than $150 per month for groceries. "You may wonder, "How does a person with a daughter survive on such a small budget?" First, we did not eat meat, and secondly, we utilized the food pantry. During this time, I learned to budget and to be thankful for my little. I also learned that I could survive by trusting God for the much-needed items (shoes, clothes, cosmetics, etc.). Many times, He provided for the additional things we desired through blessings from others or finding them on sale.

Stress Triggers Effects

According to Holmes and Rahe Stress Scale,[9] the most stressful life triggers that a person faces; is the death of loved ones and divorce, followed by moving, illness, and job loss. These emotional triggers take a toll on the body, often leading to more stress, depression, anger, anxiety, and even skin disorders. Stress releases cortisol, increasing the inflammatory response, decreasing immune response, thus interfering with the body's ability to heal.[10]

Some years back, while dealing with divorce, I experienced a high-stress level. Not understanding the process or what was happening, insomnia set in, leading to more stress, more fatigue, mental fog, and poor decision-making. The perpetual cycle lasted months, affecting my work performance, which eventually led to the loss of my job, more stress, and setbacks to paying the rent. Being in that state for a prolonged period, an itchy rash developed, covering my body. Only when my emotions stabilized did the rash disappear. However, when a high-stress event reoccurred, the itchy scaly rash resurfaced. To this day, I can tell how my body is reacting to my emotions, by how my skin responds. Thank God it does not happen too often. Note: *Not everyone's skin responds this way.*[10]

Reflection

I hope you have gained some basic knowledge of how intricate our bodies are and the importance of sleep. We all have a 24-hour day, so how we utilize. our time depends on our life goals. But no matter what, we all need adequate amounts of sleep. As you may well realize, in the wake of trying to accomplish our daily agendas, sleep is often the one area that suffers. It is not only vital for your wellbeing but for those around us. It is up to you to manage your time in such a way that you get enough sleep (young children can and often do interrupt sleep cycles). The stresses of life are not going to simply disappear. Instead, we are required to take an active role and manage our stress. A healthy diet and regular exercise can make all the difference. And since financial difficulties significantly impact our day-to-day stress levels, it would be wise to learn to manage our finances. [Note: if you are following along in the workbook, adequate sleep should be the first blocks filled in on your twenty-four-hour grid.]

Prayer

Father, I ask You to give me wisdom on what things I need to do to get a better night's sleep. I want to function at optimum in every area of my life, especially in my eating, exercising, and sleeping habits, along with my finances. I realize I may need to eliminate certain activities and break certain habits to accomplish this task. My desire is to be healthy in all areas of my life, and I need Your assistance. I thank You for this help, in Jesus' name…Amen!

2
RECHARGE AND DESTRESS

"...It is written, "Man shall not live by bread alone, but by every word that proceeds from the mouth of God" (**Matthew 4:4, NKJV**).

What happens when we Forfeit Rest?

One morning, while listening to my portable radio, suddenly the music stopped. I realized the battery was dead, and I did not have any in reserves. Battery operated technology without a power adapter or batteries will not work. We either need to recharge the batteries regularly, replace with new ones or stay continually connected to the power source. Some of us run on fumes because we fail to rest and recharge. Thus finding ourselves depleted and exhausted. I used to continually be on the go; it was difficult to sit still. My body tried to keep up with the chatter in my brain. Uncharted waters of my mind flipped from one thought to another. I was often up and out of the house early, visiting friends. I had many things going on, without any target or goal. My walk was aimless and fruitless, and I seldom said "No!"

Is it Ok to say 'No'?

Lack of rest for extended periods depletes the immune system which can produce illness. When we forfeit the overtime and take the day for rest, we may find ourselves in a better mood, more productive and less likely to become ill. We can get stressed when we take on too much, saying "Yes" to everything. We often overbook our schedules, feeling guilty if we say "No!" Since we cannot be in two places at once, we end up disappointing someone from overbooking our schedules. Over the years, I have learned to say "No!" Sometimes you must weigh the cost, extra income, or sickness from being overstressed?

In my earlier years, I did not know how to rest. I was sick more often. I attended school part-time; held several jobs; stayed up late; rarely took care of my body; and ate poorly. I didn't plan rest breaks. Most of my rest was forced, "I'm sick now, I'm taking a sick day!" There came a point in my Christian walk, where I had to slow down; plan my days; not be a Yes person; and learn to say No and be ok with it. It can be a struggle, in the beginning, to make these adjustments. Do you find yourself in this scenario…overworked, overstressed, and burnt out? Are you ready to make some changes for your physical and mental wellbeing?

Rest and Destress

I define faithful rest as a mind at peace, free from overwhelming thoughts, and having the ability to fall asleep quickly, with no worries. Taking a walk near the ocean or nature trails are naturally relaxing to me, along with the sounds of the ocean waves, a piano or soft contemporary Christian music. Other helpful ways to relax; taking an evening walk, having a bath or shower; reading a good book, drinking a cup of tea, etc.

Herbal teas are a great way to relax. It is recommended that you get direction from your physician if you are pregnant, nursing or taking certain medications. Herbal teas and supplements may cause interactions with your current medication or cause harm to the expectant mother, or fetus.[11] If you have children, you can show them how to take care of themselves by teaching them the value of quiet time. Children often incorporate the values they grow up with, and they are always watching. Therefore, they will do what you do, rather than doing what you say.

It is important to take time off to relax each week; to spend time with God, family, and friends and/or to do other things you enjoy. This frees you from burn out. There are times where I feel burnt out from the humdrum of daily living and just need a breather, I need a change of scenery to feel refreshed. Do you ever feel this way? Personally, I get bored with routine. Don't get me wrong. Having a routine is safe, predictable and most people like it, but not all people are challenged by it. We need change when things get same old, same old. Do you ever feel stagnant? Maybe it's time to change things up, to do something different. Last year, during Christmas break, I found myself needing a break from routine. During that time, I kicked up my feet, spent more time in the Word and in prayer; saw a movie; had a pedicure; and caught up on writing. My main intention was to rest in the Lord.

Do you take a day of rest each week? Or are you constantly busy, with no time for yourself or your family?

Life was not meant to go without times of refreshing. We all need rejuvenating for our souls… time away from busy schedules, work, and chores. On a regular basis, we need to break away from routines and instead, simply rest. What relaxes you? When was the last time you did something for you?

Take Time to Unwind

Taking time for yourself must be intentional. Otherwise, you may not engage. Let us think of a few things you can do. First, list things that require little or no money like taking a walk; riding a bike; going for a hike; taking the children to the park; going to the beach; walking or reading a book for 20 minutes. Make time for these activities as they are minimal in time and cost. Second, list things that are within your budget; a massage; manicure; pedicure; going to the gym; fishing; mini weekend vacation; a movie; a play;

concert in the park, etc. Schedule time for them monthly or bi-monthly. Choose things that do not cost anything, then add in something that is within your budget to do on occasion. Walking helps me destress and costs nothing but time.

Keep Your Focus

Refocusing on the Lord will give you a better perspective to what is happening around you. What helps you keep your mind and heart fixed on God? For me, reading and listening to God's Word, singing hymns and anointed worship music, praying and spending time praising God refocus my heart and mind on Him. Sometimes, it is a sacrifice to praise, especially when I do not feel like praising. Yet, in some of my most trying times, praising God until His presence showed up turned my thinking around.

Negative Thoughts

Negative thoughts that are contrary to the Word of God will whisper to your situation, "You missed God!" You may have taken every step constituting for faith, and still, you must continue to rest in His promises to bring it to fruition. Are you struggling with these kinds of thoughts? It is time to lean more on God and spend more time in His presence and in His Word. It is time to find that place where you can rest, knowing that God is an on-time God. It's not over until God says it's over; there is a song I like to sing,

> "He's an on-time God, yes He is! He is an on-time God, Yes, He is! He may not come when you want Him, but He'll be there right on time, I'll tell you, He's an on-time God, yes He is!"
> (Dottie Peoples).[12]

Reflection

It is time to take back your schedule with a plan. If you do not have a plan for your time, it is easy to ride the waves saying "Yes" to everything. Taking on too much will only increase your stress level and make you ineffective. A carefully planned schedule will allow you the time to get important things done while allowing time to care for family and yourself. When you are less stressed, you are less negative, and it is a win-win for everyone.

Prayer

Father help me to take back my life with a schedule and plan. I know at times I need to be flexible, however, I've been saying "yes" to things when I really need to say "no!" I know your word says, "But let your 'Yes' be 'Yes,' and your 'No,' 'No', For whatever is more than these is from the evil one" (**Matthew 5:37 NKJV**). You know the plans you have for me. I ask that you give me direction for my days, and that I spend my time wisely doing those things that will profit the plans you have for me. I ask you to help me balance my life in such a way that I can make time for all the things that are important in my life. I ask this in Jesus's name…Amen!

3
BIBLICAL REST

"Every person needs to take one day away. A day in which one consciously separates the past from the future. Jobs, family, employers, and friends can exist one day without any one of us, and if our egos permit us to confess, they could exist eternally in our absence. Each person deserves a day away in which no problems are confronted, no solutions searched for. Each of us needs to withdraw from the cares which will not withdraw from us" (Maya Angelou,
Wouldn't Take Nothing for My Journey
Now).[13]

In the Beginning

God took a world that was dark and void and created the foundation by which the next phase of life could be sustained. The Bible tells us in

Genesis 1:3-5,

> "And on the seventh day God ended His work which He had done, and He rested on the seventh day from all His work which He had done" (NKJV).

Then God said, "Let there be light…So the evening and the morning were the first day. On the second day, God created the firmament and called it the sky and divided the waters from the sky, calling the sky heaven. On the third day, God gathered the waters together and made the dry land appear. "He called the dry land Earth, and the gathering together of the waters He called Seas. And God saw that it was good." Then God said, "Let the earth bring forth grass, the herb that yields seed, and the fruit tree that yields fruit according to

its kind, whose seed is in itself on the earth."
And all that God said transpired and God
said, "it was good." On the fourth day, God
made the skies, sun, stars, and moon to "be for
signs and seasons." The sun to rule the day
and the moon and stars to rule the night.

On the fifth day, God created the birds and sea
creatures and commanded they become
fruitful and multiply according to their kind.
On the sixth day, God created the land animals
and every other kind of creeping creature, and
they abounded according to their kind."

Now that the foundational elements for life
were abundant, and man's DNA inspired, life
could be sustained continually. God had
provided every element to sustain the earth,
man, and every living creature: mineral
nutrients; water; trees for oxygen and shelter;
animals for food and herbs; and plants for
medicinal purposes.

Then God tells man, "I give you dominion
over every living thing. Be fruitful and
multiply. This was the sixth day.

On the seventh day, God rested from all that He created. He had completed all that was needed to sustain life. God had set the foundation and the pattern by which man shall live; work six days creating with your hands, providing food for your families, and on the seventh day, rest.

Exodus 23:12,

> "Six days you shall do your work, and on the seventh day you shall rest, that your ox and your donkey may rest, and the son of your female servant and the stranger may be refreshed" (NKJV).

God made provision for all living creatures, including the animals that labored alongside man in the fields. They, too, needed rest and refreshment.

Define Rest

In the Bible, there are two meanings for rest. First, to rest from one's labors. Its Hebrew meaning, "nuach,[14]" to rest, to be quiet, often synonymous with Shabbat; to cease or to rest.

In Greek, this same "rest" is defined as cessation or refreshment, "anapausis."[15] In **Hebrews 10:11-14,** the priests are ministering daily, offering the same sacrifices repeatedly, which can never take away sins. (But our High Priest offered himself to God as a single sacrifice for sins, good for all time. Then he sat down in the place of honor at God's right hand). In the first part of this scripture, we see the priest standing and ministering daily. They were working continually for something that did not produce eternal results. Standing continually places strain, not only on the body but the mind. It zaps your energy. But Jesus on the other hand, finished His work, afterward sitting down. When I think of sitting down, I think of resting. And that is Jesus' stance…He sits from a place of rest, waiting for His enemies to become His footstool.

However, there was another kind of rest. A rest that encompassed Faith and trust in Jehovah God. In the Old Testament, the

Israelites continually complained of God's provision in the wilderness. They failed to enter their Promised Land (a place of rest and provision) because of their unbelief, hardened hearts, and disobedience. Thus, they walked around in the wilderness, going around the same mountains for forty years (kind of like men today).

What mountains have you found yourself going around repeatedly? Are you ready to address these mountains?

Psalm 95

King David says:

> "Oh come, let us sing to the Lord! Let us shout joyfully to the Rock of our salvation. Let us come before His presence with thanksgiving; Let us shout joyfully to Him with psalms. For the Lord is the great God, And the great King above all gods. In His hand are the deep places of the earth; The heights of the hills are His also. The sea is His, for

He made it; And His hands formed the dry land. Oh come, let us worship and bow down; Let us kneel before the Lord our Maker. For He is our God, and we are the people of His pasture, And the sheep of His hand. Today, if you will hear His voice: Do not harden your hearts as in the rebellion, As in the day of trial in the wilderness. When your fathers tested Me; They tried Me, though they saw My work. For forty years I was grieved with that generation, And said, 'It is a people who go astray in their hearts, and they do not know My ways.' So, I swore in My wrath, 'They shall not enter My rest,'" (NKJV) referred to as the land of promise (Amp), God's ultimate blessings (NLT).

Workaholism

Exodus 34:21,

"Six days you shall work, but on the seventh day you shall rest; in plowing

time and in harvest you shall rest"
(NKJV).

Today, high performers are a valued commodity. They are focused, proactive, successful, and know how to implement their goals, and can balance work, family, and recreation. On the other hand, workaholics tend to lack focus, work excessively, and alienate co-workers, family, and recreation. They are perfectionists at best, unable to meet even their own high standards. They often suffer from insomnia, anxiety, anger, fear, or depression. Their busyness is often a cover-up to avoid facing their feelings or some other underlying cause, such as insecurity. To avoid facing their unpleasant feelings they may have grown up with, such as both parents being workaholics (driven by a compulsion to work), they rarely find time off refreshing. Matter of fact, resting is difficult.

Workaholism is defined as "an addiction to work, the compulsion and uncontrollable need to work incessantly."[14] Workaholism, like any other addiction, has negative ramifications. It is often overlooked as a problem today. While employers' value a hard worker, they often find that workaholism interferes with work performance.[17]

Are you a workaholic? How does it affect others in your life (For better or for worse)? Are you willing to adjust your schedule to bring healing to your relationships?

A Day of Rest

Usually on Saturday until Sunday from late afternoon, I take a day off for rest, including taking a break from my school studies. Saturday nights are often (but not always) movie nights, then I spend Sunday mornings with my church family, visit my mom in the afternoon, then go home. Sometimes, I take a nap. Afterward, I feel refreshed and relaxed, taking the remainder of Sunday to prepare for the week.

When was the last time you consciously took a full day of rest? How did you feel afterward?

Do you do this on a regular basis? If you could, would you do this every week? If it

made you more productive, would you, do it? What is stopping you from taking one full day off to be with God and with your family, to have some fun together?

Reflection

For some, Friday is the end of the workweek. [Thank God It's Friday (T.G.I.F.)]. Those who are ready for the weekend may not find resting difficult. However, for others, they work throughout the week, and now they have the responsibility of keeping up the internal and external areas of the home. Remember the word of God, six days you shall work, and on the seventh day, you shall rest.

Work is a responsibility we must carry. The Bible says in

2 Thessalonians 3:10,

> "For even when we were with you, we commanded you this: 'If anyone will not work, neither shall he eat" (NKJV).

But God laid the pattern through His own actions, that the seventh day would not be complete without a day of rest. You may work on Saturday and Sunday, as I know many people who work in healthcare do. When I worked in healthcare, at one point, I remember praying to God, asking Him to make a way for me to have Sundays off to attend church. Amazingly, He made away. Even so, you can dedicate another day during the week for rest, even honoring God with that day by spending time with Him in the Word.

Prayer

Father, thank You for providing the work of my hands, blessing my bread and butter, and meeting all my needs, according to your riches in Glory. I want to honor You and my family by taking one day a week to rest from work. Lord, you got all Your work done in six days and then rested, showing me the pattern for which to model. Father help me arrange my schedule in such a way that I get my work done in six days, so I can honor You and my body with rest each week. In Jesus' name, I pray, Amen!

4
REST FOR THE SOUL

"God's grace is the healing sustenance for
the soul."[21]

Trusting God Brings Rest

Have you ever faced troubles that should have caused unrest but instead you had peace?

Philippians 4:7 says,

> "and the peace of God, which surpasses all understanding, will guard your hearts and minds through Christ Jesus" (NKJV).

When you have peace in situations that would make the 'worldly Joe' anything but peaceful, that's God! There is a place in God given to those who trust in Him and fix their eyes on the Lord. That place is revealed in **Psalm 91**

> "…the secret place of the Most-High" (NKJV).

In 2014, the Lord led me to meditate on **Psalm 91,** of which many are acquainted with. I put the psalm to memory by reading it repeatedly, incorporating it into a personal prayer for myself and others. Here, I found solace as I meditated on trusting God.

Putting the Past to Rest

Entering God's rest must be settled within. As a man struggles with weakness, a studied man always goes back to the Word of God, asking himself the questions: Am I aligning my behavior and actions to God's Word? Am I resting in His truths, His promises?

I found myself at times struggling with my schedule. So much needed to get done, yet I find it difficult to incorporate it all. I was worse on myself than God was on me. We are often our own worst critics, aren't we? If the Lord requires that we be flexible, isn't He then also flexible? God is not rigid with pettiness. Isn't it like the devil to portray God as a taskmaster? And isn't it like a man to believe God is a rigid and overbearing tyrant, ready to smack us down for every little mistake?

My dad was raised Methodist; my grandmother was strict with him. He taught

Sunday school until he was 18, but after high school and upon entering the army, he stopped. His desire for the army was to be a helicopter pilot. However, because he lacked 20/20 vision, he was unable to pilot. Instead, he was trained by the army in electrical engineering. He spent the remainder of his career working on the space program at the Space Center on the east coast of Florida.

Growing up, my parents never took me to church together. Up until I was 6, my mom took me and my older sister to the Methodist church. She would drop me off at Sunday school, then head to the adult building with the stained-glass windows. On our yearly visits to grandma's house, I often heard my dad and my grandma in heated discussions, but I was too young to understand. The only thing that stayed in my memory was hearing them argue over politics and God.

My grandmother's threats, "Henry, if you don't stop, you're going to end up in hell!" My dad would spat back, "If God is such a mean God, I don't want to serve Him!" Those arguments rung in my ears for most of my life. My entire family was turned off by my grandmother's harsh judgments and rigid rules, which repelled them from God. Even so, Dad was faithful to take us to visit our extended family in Georgia every year. After age 6, my mom no longer took us to church, but my parents never kept me or my sister from learning about God. They gave us permission to go to church every Sunday on the Baptist Church bus, and other times with friends. We both attended church into our mid-teens. My dad professed a more liberal viewpoint, deciding he was a humanist. Even so, I often saw him watching Christian programs. He kept a Bible in the house, which I referenced on occasion. In my teen years, I began to have a mixed view of God. My dad a proclaimed atheist, myself a confused agnostic; not believing what my dad professed, yet, not quite sure where God fitted into my life. Although I did not know, at the time, I had been given a warped view of God.

From age 16 to 24, I lived a life absent from church. Then in 1993, I was introduced to a few people who, unknowingly at the time, were the light of Jesus in my dark world. In March of 1998, I gave my life to Christ. One day, while leaving my parents' house, my dad remarked, "If I turned back now, I would be a hypocrite." By then, he had already been diagnosed with cancer (twice), mouth cancer, and Non-Hodgkin's lymphoma. I was still a babe in Christ, and although I knew what my dad meant, I did not know how to deal with that statement. In November of 1998, my husband and I moved to Connecticut. Since I had left Florida, I had not been plugged into a church, or the Word of God. Thus, I was not growing in my walk with the Lord. My dad had been stable for the remainder of 1998 and 1999, but in 2000, he was diagnosed with metastatic lung cancer. Meanwhile, my husband and I were rejoicing in the new life that was growing on the inside. My dad had been desiring a grandchild. It was a difficult time, yet it was the very thing that drew me back to God. Easter 2000, I rededicated my life to the Lord.

At the end of May 2000, my dad was scheduled for a left lung lobectomy. During the surgery they found contraindications that prevented them from removing the lung. Post-surgery went well, so it seemed until things turned for the worse. Since he could not breathe on his own, he was taken to ICU, where he was hooked up to a ventilator for a few days to see if it could be reversed. By this time, I was seven months pregnant. At this stage in my pregnancy, it was not advisable to fly. However, my doctor gave me permission. Upon arrival, my family and I went to the hospital to visit my dad. My sister and I went into the room to say our goodbyes since he decided not to stay on the ventilator. Because of the agitation, he was highly medicated. With my sister on one side, and me on the other, I took his hand, but immediately he jerked away. My sister spoke while I sat at his side, unable to say a word. It was the most heart-wrenching time of my life. I could not escape the room fast enough. All that rang in my head was where was his soul going after death! Where was he going to spend eternity! All the conversations of what he believed and did not believe flashed across my mind. All the conversations of my grandma's judgmental remarks! The time he was afraid of being a hypocrite! I could not get any of it out of my head, and this haunted me for years! I did not know, and it scared me!

Three years later in 2003, during a relationship crisis, all my misconstrued beliefs about God flooded to the surface, leaving me anxious and paralyzed by an unhealthy fear of God. Then in 2009, I questioned the Lord about my dad's eternal home. It brought me much turmoil. As part of the healing process, I needed to come to a place of rest. I sensed the Lord saying, "Put it to rest." Once I had peace in my soul that he was OK, I was able to let go and move on. Since then, the Lord has graciously taught me about His grace. Even revealing, as judgmental as my grandmother was, there was grace and rest for her soul. God knows how to keep those who truly belong to Him. Who are (we to say) whom God speaks to on their death bed?

Psalm 89:30-33 says,

"If his sons forsake My law and do not walk in My judgments, if they break My statutes And do not keep My commandments, Then I will punish their transgression with the rod, And their iniquity with stripes. Nevertheless, My lovingkindness I will not utterly take from him, Nor allow My faithfulness to fail" (NKJV).

This is our God! Faithful, loving, kind, yet just in His judgments!

Reflection

Who do you turn to when you are struggling? Do you go to God or someone else? Are there things from your past that you need healing from and need to lay to rest? God can lead you to a healing place. It might not happen as quickly as you would like, but if you ask Him, and follow His leading, He will.

Prayer

Father, my past is continually causing me unrest. Today, I want to lay them at Your feet (list those things you need to lay to rest). Father God, I ask You to lead me down this healing journey, that I will make the necessary changes and receive the peace that surpasses all understanding. Teach me Your ways, that I may trust You, and draw closer to You. I ask this in Jesus, name. Amen.

5
A SHEMITAH REST

"Shemitah demonstrates that the earth needs to rest as an ecological necessity, just as people need to rest as a spiritual necessity. Shemitah represents an ideal, an expanded perspective which seeks out meaning in all experiences and moves us to treat the world around us, and its fruits, with the sanctity they deserve."[22]

Carbon and Nitrogen are two of the six essential life-sustaining elements known to living organisms. "Together, they account for almost 98 percent of Earth's living matter"[23]. They are especially vital to the soil we use to grow our food. Carbon produces carbon dioxide, a product needed for photosynthesis and carbohydrate production. Nitrogen makes proteins for amino acids, the building blocks of cells, and carbohydrates for energy.[24] This second element demonstrates how essential healthy soil is to our crops. Remove one building block, and the process of life disrupts.

Isaiah 55:10

> "For as the rain comes down, and the snow from heaven, And do not return there, but water the earth, And make it bring forth and bud, That it may give seed to the sower And bread to the eater" (NKJV).

Under Hebrew law, upon the Israelites entering Canaan, their "promised land," were required to honor God and the land through a Shemitah. A Shemitah year, according to Strong's Concordance is a year of "remission, remittance," to temporarily cease from working the land. A Shemitah year, also known as a Sabbatical year, occurred every seventh year. A year of rest for the land.[25]

Each, forty-nine years, would be followed by a Jubilee. In the fiftieth year, debts (were canceled) and slaves set free. Those who did not honor the Shemitah, or seventh year, by letting the land lay fallow were exiled. Either way, the ground would get its rest, either through obedience or by consequences thereof. For every "Shemitah," they failed to let the land rest (490 years), the Lord sent them into exile (70 years).[25]

God knew what He was doing when He
declared a sabbath rest for the land.

Leviticus 25:2-5,

> "…When you come into the land which I
> give you, then the land shall keep a
> sabbath to the Lord. Six years you shall
> sow your field, and six years you shall
> prune your vineyard, and gather its
> fruit; but in the seventh year, there shall
> be a sabbath of solemn rest for the land,
> a sabbath to the Lord. You shall neither
> sow your field nor prune your vineyard.
> What grows of its own accord of your
> harvest you shall not reap, nor gather
> the grapes of your untended vine, for it
> is a year of rest for the land" (NKJV).

**"Take rest; a field that has rested gives a
beautiful crop"[26]**

Agriculture was a significant aspect of
antiquity culture. By law, farmers had to plant
their land and vineyards for six years, but

every seventh year, they had to let the land lay fallow. There were a few reasons for this.

- **First,** the farmers had to leave the land untouched, allowing it to produce whatever it yielded that year.
- **Second,** they would allow only the animals to roam the land, fertilizing it during that year. This process would replenish the soil, bringing the right elemental mix.
- **Third,** whatever the fallow land produced (on its own) was left for the poor to glean.[27]

Farmers understand that the nourishment of the soil matters. But over time, men have become greedy, depleting the nutrients of the soil through continual planting.

Winter is also a time for the land to rest and replenish its nutrients. Well rested and nutrient-rich, the earth becomes increasingly fertile.[27] In a sense, we have laid fallow in the season of Covid-19, an unexpected, forced rest.

Many have even chuckled at the thought that more babies would be born in November and December of 2020.

What happens to a land that receives a sabbath rest?

A land that does not get its rest yields more harmful insects that degrade the soil, causing water run-off versus water absorption conducive to a land well-rested. Furthermore, when the farmland can rest from continual growth, as God intended, there is no need for fertilizers and chemicals. Letting the land rest will restore nutrient-rich soil through increase carbon stores, thus producing a better yield of fruits and vegetables.[28]

The Covid-19 pandemic of 2020 caught the world off guard, overtaken by an unseen enemy, the SARS (Severe Acute Respiratory Syndrome) virus from Wuhan China. It spread quickly, with many unknowns about its pathology and etiology. The solution to prevent its spread led many nations to quarantine some areas over a month. What impact or implication does that have on rest? Within a short time, airline travel ceased; cities across the world shut down; cities that never sleep, like New York City, were empty.

In just a short time, people around the world made some unusual discoveries. In northern India, the people noted that they could see the Himalaya Mountains, something they had not witnessed in thirty years.[29] In Venice, Italy, with motorboats and cars parked due to the shutdown, people noticed better air quality and clearer water canals, something the people had not experienced in years.[30] Also, with Los Angeles highways and byways empty for over a month, residents noted better air quality, along with no visible signs of smog.[31]

Furthermore, emissions were down in China, with fewer cars on the streets. So much so, the country noted a forty percent decrease in the fuel byproduct, Nitrogen dioxide. These were significant changes to the environment during quarantine 2020.[32] Although only temporary, these were remarkable improvements to our environment with a little rest from the hand of man.

Reflection

When a man honors God's creation by tending to it, taking what he needs, and obeying the natural laws God instituted from the beginning; everyone wins. However, many people are filled with greed, thinking only of their immediate needs and not the long-term implications from overuse of the land. Do you think God changed His mind about how to properly farm the earth so that it produces the proper elemental mix? The latest inventions are to make things easier on man, but over the years, we have found, instead, that they have harmed our environment. Even though Covid-19 brought much uncertainty, it certainly shined the light on man's contribution to the constant overuse of resources and what a little consistent rest could do.

Prayer

Father forgive me for my greed in wanting to meet only my immediate needs without thinking of the long-term implications of my overuse of natural resources such as water, electricity, fuel, and food. Help me to become a better steward over all that You have given me. I ask this, in Jesus' name, Amen.

6
OUTCOMES FROM LACK OF REST

"Let us then give diligence, that we may have a clear entrance into the kingdom of God. As God finished his work, and then rested from it, so he will cause those who believe, to finish their work, and then to enjoy their rest"[33]

Psalm 95:8-10,

> "Do not harden your hearts, as in the rebellion, as in the day of trial in the wilderness, When your fathers tested Me; They tried Me, though they saw My work. For forty years I was grieved with that generation (first generation of Israelis), And said, 'It is a people who go astray in their hearts, And they do not know My ways. So I swore in My wrath, 'They shall not enter My rest'" (NKJV).

God has a rest for His people, and He wants us to enter His rest, but not everyone who says "Lord, Lord" will enter God's rest. Why? First because of unbelief, which is defined as incredulity or skepticism, especially in matters of religious faith. Those with unbelief do not believe in God and His Word. Secondly, for Hardness of Heart. Synonyms for Hardness of Heart are animosity; antagonism; enmity; grudge; hatred; bitterness; harshness; hostility; ill will; resentful; aversion; spite; variance; vengeful and uncharitable,[34] to name a few.

Their hearts are hardened by the cares of this world.

Lastly because of Disobedience to God's Word. Disobedience, according to the *Dictionary*, is defined as a lack of obedience or refusal to comply, disregard, or transgression.[35]

Hebrews 4:1-10,

"Therefore, since a promise remains of entering His rest, let us fear lest any of you seem to have come short of it. For indeed the gospel was preached to us as well as to them; but the word which they heard did not profit them, not being mixed with faith in those who heard it. For we who have believed do enter that rest, as He has said: "So I swore in My wrath, 'They shall not enter My rest,' "although the works were finished from the foundation of the world. For He has spoken in a certain place of the seventh day in this way: "And God rested on the seventh day from all His works;" and again in this place: "They shall not enter My rest." Since therefore it remains that some must enter it, and those to whom it was first preached did not enter because of disobedience, again He designates a certain day, saying in David, "Today,"after such a long time, as it has been said: "Today, if you will hear His voice, Do not harden your hearts. "For if Joshua had given them rest, then He would not afterward have spoken of another day. There remains therefore a rest for the people of God. For he who has entered His rest has himself also ceased from his works as God did from His."[36]

Who are examples of those who did not enter God's rest? Why didn't they enter God's rest?

Moses and Aaron did not enter the Promised Land because they failed to follow the instruction of the Lord.

"Then the Lord spoke to Moses, saying, 'Take the rod; you and your brother Aaron gather the congregation together. Speak to the rock before their eyes, and it will yield its water; thus, you shall bring water for them out of the rock and give drink to the congregation and their animals. 'So, Moses took the rod from before the Lord as He commanded him. And Moses and Aaron gathered the assembly together before the rock; and he said to them, 'Hear now, you rebels! Must we bring water for you out of this rock?' Then Moses lifted his hand and struck the rock twice with his rod; and water came out abundantly, and the congregation and their animals drank. Then the Lord spoke to Moses and Aaron, 'Because you did not believe Me, to hallow Me in the eyes of the children of Israel, therefore you shall not bring this assembly into the land which I have given them (NKJV).'"

By not following the Lord's set of instructions, Moses and Aaron dishonored God. God told them to "speak to the rock before their eyes, and it will yield its water," but instead, Moses scolded the congregation and struck the rock twice, "Hear now, you rebels!" Although God gave water from the rock, there were ramifications for the brothers' disobedience. As leaders, God held them to a higher standard. Thus, due to their disobedience Moses, Aaron, and the Israelites (because of their continual grumbling and complaining) failed to enter the Promised Land. God was bringing them to their inheritance.

Deuteronomy 12:8-10,

> "You shall not at all do as we are doing here today…every man doing whatever is right in his own eyes…for as yet you have not come to the rest and the inheritance which the Lord your God is giving you. But when you cross over the Jordan and dwell in the land where the Lord your God is giving you to inherit, and He gives you rest from all your

enemies round about, so that you dwell in safety… then there will be the place where the Lord your God chooses to make His name abide" (NKJV).

"Christ had works to do, preaching the Gospel, performing miracles, and obtaining the redemption and salvation of his people: these were given him to do, and he undertook them, and he has finished them; and so ceases from them, as never to repeat them more; they being done effectually, stand in no need of it; and so as to take delight and complacency in them; the pleasure of the Lord prospering in, his hand, the effects of his labor answering his designs; just as God ceased from the works of creation, when he had finished them"[35]

Things to Lay to Rest

Hebrews 12:1,

"Therefore, since we are surrounded by such a huge crowd of witnesses to the life of faith, let us strip off every weight that slows us down, especially the sin that so easily trips us up. And let us run with endurance the race God has set before us" (NLT).

What things are weighing you down? Are you a grumbler and complainer-- never satisfied with anything? This may be a weight that is hindering your walk of faith. Remember the Israelites wandered in the wilderness for forty years (when they could have been resting in their promised land), all because of their constant complaining. Are there areas in your own life that interfere with your obedience to God? What are the sins that repeatedly trip you up? List them. Ask the Lord to forgive you, then thank Him for His mercy and grace to help you overcome in these areas.

To counter the bad habit of grumbling and complaining, I have found that being intentionally grateful helps. When the focus is on the blessings, no matter how little or big, our mindset changes from grumbling to an attitude of gratitude and thanksgiving. This pleases the Lord.

Reflection

Many need to gain wisdom from the Word of God. We believe in God but fail to study the

Word to show ourselves approved, rightly dividing the Word of truth. Therefore, we are often skeptical, falling into unbelief. The world is filled with harshness and bitterness; thus, we must wash ourselves by spending time in the Word. Being doers of the Word is important to safeguard our hearts from bitterness. Only the Lord knows how to soften our hearts and keep them pliable, but we must first choose to yield to Him and walk in His will.

Prayer

Father forgive me for all my grumbling and complaining. When I look at my life, I can see that I am truly blessed. I thank You for this day! I thank You for the roof over my head, the clothes on my back. I thank You for my arms, my legs, and the ability to get up and walk. I thank You for my family and friends. I

thank You that I have a job and I thank You for
the future jobs You have for me, I thank You
for providing food on my table. I thank You
for health, eyes to see, ears to hear and the
ability to think. I thank You for sending Your
Son Jesus, who saved me from my sins and
eternal separation from You…I thank You that
I can have a relationship with You…and that
You give me guidance and direction, leading
me into paths of righteousness…for with You I
am truly blessed! In Jesus' name…Amen!

7
TRUST GOD

"Worrying is carrying tomorrow's load with today's strength- carrying two days at once. It is moving into tomorrow ahead of time. Worrying doesn't empty tomorrow of its sorrow, it empties today of its strength"[37]

Romans 10:17,

> "So, then faith comes by hearing, and hearing by the word of God" (NKJV).

There are times in our lives where we experience a delay. When this happens, we need to remind ourselves that delays do not necessarily mean denial. God's encompassing presence is our safety net at such times. It helps to keep our minds continually fixed on Him. If we remain in His presence, our faith will be unwavering. But life happens, and as we sludge through each day, we may need to refocus our attention on the Lord. Refocusing on the Lord will give us a better perspective.

In Acts 16 we learn that Paul had wanted to go to Asia to preach the word, but for some reason, the Holy Spirit led him to Macedonia instead. The Bible does not say why Paul was forbidden. It could have been for his protection or any other reason, but in the end, he was not denied. He was rerouted and eventually led back to Asia.

Acts 19:10,

> "…so that all who dwelt in Asia heard the word of the Lord Jesus, both Jews and Greeks" (NKJV).

Even though your dreams have yet to be realized, keep on dreaming, and press ahead. Rest in God's promise to bring it to fruition.

Philippians 1:6,

> "…being confident of this very thing, that He who has begun a good work in you will complete it until the day of Jesus Christ…" (NKJV).

"Pray, and let God worry"[38]

Have you ever found yourself on the perpetual wheel of worry? Fifteen years ago, the Lord shined a light on my worrisome thoughts. He revealed the constant noise in my mind. It never occurred to me, until that moment, how much I worried. I wasn't restful about anything; my thought patterns were a mess. One night while extremely restless and unable to sleep, I cried out, "Lord, why can't I sleep?" Immediately, a thought came to mind, "You are not in faith; you are not trusting Me; you are not resting." Worry had consumed my thoughts. A "me" moment! Realizing my sin, I quickly repented, asking the Lord to forgive me for my lack of faith. In an instant, my mind went from turmoil to peace. I could have had peace hours earlier. However, I never talked to God about the situation. I just mulled over it. Why did it take so long to ask God for guidance? The dividing line was repenting of worry and asking God for assistance. "Ok Lord, I need Your wisdom."

I would like to say that was the end of the lesson, however, within minutes, I went back to worrying. I needed a lot of grace that night, as it took a couple of tries to relinquish worry. When I finally let go, I was able to rest in God and fall asleep.

Have you ever worried so much you couldn't sleep? Bad habits are often a challenge to break and even harder to recognize. Next time you find yourself unable to sleep because of worry, acknowledge what you are worrying about. Then ask the Lord to forgive you and seek His wisdom. It may take a few attempts, but with practice, it will become a good habit.

Casting your Worries

A minister friend of mine once explained "worry" this way: It's like casting your fishing line out as far as you can, knowing eventually it will draw near, and you will have to cast it out again. That is how thoughts are; we must continually cast worrying thoughts away from us. The next time you find yourself worrying, do what **1 Peter 5:7** says,

"casting all your care upon Him, for He cares for you" (NKJV).

Release Your Heavy Burdens

Matthew 11:28-30,

> "Come to Me, all you who labor and are
> heavy laden, and I will give you rest.
> Take My yoke upon you and learn from
> Me, for I am gentle and lowly in heart,
> and you will find rest for your souls. For
> My yoke is easy and my burden is light"
> (NKJV).

A yoke is a harness used to separate a pair of
oxen as they plow a plot of land. Since the
land was often hardened from the winter, it
took a sharp plow to dig deep into the earth to
break up the hardened ground. Together, two
oxen could carry a heavier load. The owner
steered the oxen as the oxen plowed and tilled
the land.

Servants who had been yoked to tyrant rulers
were oppressed and heavy laden. Their yoke
was not easy. As slaves to these oppressive

leaders, the Israelites often carried extremely heavy objects (burdens) upon their bodies.

Jesus beckons those who are heavily laden, with the weight of the world, to come to Him.

He assured them that if they came into His Kingdom, they would be treated with gentleness, humility, and respect, versus the oppressive rule they were under. In such a switch, they would have rest for their souls.[40]

Heavy Loads

Many people are tired and weary of all the racial injustice going on in America. Over and over, black men and women of God are saying, "I'm tired, when will racism end?" Mothers are concerned for the welfare of their Black sons. A mother (I heard) expresses her son coming to the rightful age of 16, to obtain his driving permit, but faced with the reality that he may be a product of racial profiling. Do you have heavy burdens you need to lay at the feet of Jesus? Jesus beckons you to cast your care upon Him. Lay it at His feet. He will help you carry the loads in life if you ask Him. Call upon Him and let Him relieve you and refresh you.

Resting in God's Timing

Although our dreams and desires may not transpire as planned, it does not mean the dream will not materialize. At times, my imagination gets the best of me, causing disappointment for having to go around the same mountain repeatedly.

Disappointment happens when we do not give room for flexibility, detours, and roadblocks. The journey to our dreams is not always foreseeable. We must leave room for alternative routes. We must assess the possibilities and be ready to adjust and accept a different outcome. The important thing is to be flexible, to adapt, and to proceed. Keep believing that the Lord is working it out!

Even though we may wrestle within, resting in God's will and timing for our lives can help decrease inner turmoil. It takes time to get acquainted with God and to hear His still, small voice.

Reflection

Learning to cast our care upon the Lord does not always happen overnight. It is often a battle of our will, and we must take intentional strides to break through to a place of rest. When we seek God for wisdom and direction during our struggles, even during the setbacks and detours, we win. Are you ready to lay your heavy burdens at the feet of Jesus?

Prayer

Dear Father, I have been worried about many things (name them) lately, and today I humbly come to You and ask You to help me lay these burdens at your feet. I ask for Your wisdom and direction. You know what is best for me, and I trust You, Lord, knowing You will lead me in the paths of righteousness. Most of all, I want to follow Your will and Your plan for my life. Help me to hear Your voice, follow Your instructions, and be flexible to Your leading. I am resting my care upon You. I ask all of this, in Jesus' name…Amen!

EPILOGUE

Acts 3:19 states,

> "Repent therefore and be converted, that your sins may be blotted out, so that times of refreshing may come from the presence of the Lord" (NKJV).

As we have determined, adequate sleep is an important function for optimum health. Furthermore, we must remember that as humans we are more than physical bodies. We must also attend to and feed our spiritual health. Resting in the Lord in quiet and solitude is a significant part of our spiritual well-being. Many times, we are overrun by the noise of life and have difficulty settling in silence. If we sit long enough, we may realize the constant noise of our brain.

If you have never sat still for 15 minutes without TV, people, animals, phone, or other interruptions, you may find yourself unable to settle a busy mind. Realizing this for the first time was overwhelming for me, sitting still with God for five minutes was a challenge. I heard (for the first time) the constant chatter of my mind and wished it would be silent. But that is where I started…five minutes…then gradually and over time, I have learned to sit longer in silence, with my focus on Him.

Rest…You Win is God's reminder to His body of believers, to take care of themselves. Many people are worn out from the cares of life and overwork. They do not know how to deal with the stress and therefore, live on the perpetual wheel of emotional and physical depletion. That is the time to slow down, eat better, and take time every week for God and your family.

Rest comes from a right relationship with God. We enter that relationship by believing in our hearts and confessing with our mouth that Jesus is Lord!

1 Corinthians 12:3,

> "…no one can say Jesus is Lord except by
> the Holy Spirit" (NKJV).

After the initial act of receiving Him by faith, we will begin to establish a relationship with Christ. As we develop an intimate relationship with the triune God: Father, Son, and Spirit, the Holy Spirit begins to teach us through His word.

Apart from Christ, there is no rest. Once we complete God's work here on earth, we will receive our reward for our loyalty to Him and enter the rest God prepared for us.

Most importantly, those who have accepted Jesus as their Lord and Savior, have an eternal rest for their souls. Remember, Rest…You Win!

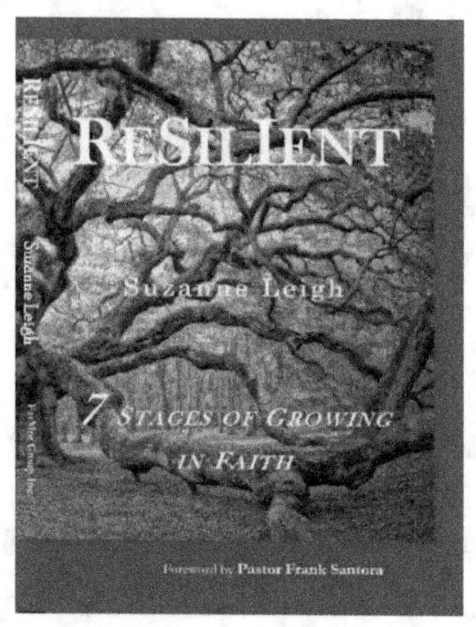

Scan the QR code to go directly to Amazon for the purchase of all books.

Rest…You Win Workbook available for download Aug. 2021 @ www.suzanneleigh.org

To contact or keep up with current and future writing and speaking engagements, please visit www.suzanneleigh.org

Works Cited

Introduction

[1]Merriam-Webster Incorp. "Rest." *Merriam-Webster*, Merriam-Webster, 2020, www.merriamwebster.com/dictionary/rest.
[2]"Stress Symptoms: Physical Effects of Stress on the Body." *WebMD*, WebMD, 1 Aug. 2019, www.webmd.com/balance/stressmanagement/stress-symptoms-effects_of-stress-onthe-body.

Chapter 1 Rest for the Body

Psalm 127:2 NIV, Proverbs 3:24 NIV, Ecclesiastes 2:23 (NASB)

[3]American Psychological Association. "Why Sleep Is Important." *American Psychological Association*, American Psychological Association, May 2020, www.apa.org/topics/sleep/why.

[4]US Dept of Transportation. "What Are the DOT Regulations for Trucks?" *Reference*, IAC Publishing, 2019, www.reference.com/article/dotregulations-trucks-1088fb70bee692c?aq=dot%2Btruck%2Bregula tions &qo=cdpArticles.

[5]Health Prep. "Warning Signs of Sleep Deprivation." *Warning Signs Of Sleep Deprivation - HealthPrep.com*, May 2016, healthprep.com/topics/sleep-disorders/warningsigns-sleep-deprivation/?xcid=3363&utm_source=bing&ut m_m edium=ppc-F1063MYF&utm_campaign=370295645&utm _cont ent=1260040937856576&utm_term=what%2 Bhapp ens%2Bif%2Byou%2Bhave%2Black%2Bof% 2Bsle ep&msclkid=28a03ebe8d081e5f89f2606bacac 4341

[6]Premier Health. "Beware High Levels of Cortisol, the Stress Hormone." *Premier Health*, May 2017, www.premierhealth.com/yourhealth/articles/women-wisdom-wellness-/bewarehigh-levels-of-cortisol-the-stress-hormone.

[7]Berkley, Cherie. "What You Eat Can Sabotage Your Sleep." *WebMD*, WebMD, 2019, www.webmd.com/sleep-disorders/features/foodsabotage-sleep#1.

[8]Brainy Quote. "Suze Orman Quotes." *BrainyQuote*, Xplore, 2020, www.brainyquote.com/quotes/suze_orman_173481.

[9]Briggs, Myers, et al. "10 Most Stressful Life Events: the Holmes and Rahe Stress Scale." *Pain Doctor*, 14

Mar. 2018, paindoctor.com/top-10-stressful-lifeevents-holmes-rahe-stress-scale/.

[10]Harvard Health Publishing. "Recognizing the MindSkin Connection." *Harvard Health*, Nov. 2006,www.health.harvard.edu/newsletter_article/Recogni zing_the_mind-skin_connection.

Chapter 2 Recharge and Destress

Matthew 4:4, NKJV, Matthew 5:37, NKJV

[11]Anderson, Leigh Ann. "18 Herbal Supplements with Risky Drug Interactions." *Drugs.com*, 2020, www.drugs.com/slideshow/herb-drug-interactions1069.

[12]"He`s An On Time God - Dottie Peoples." *SongLyrics.com*, 2020, www.songlyrics.com/dottiepeoples/he-s-an-on-time-god-lyrics/.

Chapter 3 Biblical Rest

Genesis 1:35, NKJV, Exodus 23:12, NKJV, Hebrews
10:11-14, Psalm 95, NKJV, 2 Thessalonians 3:10, NKJV

[13]Goodreads. "A Quote from Wouldn't Take Nothing for My Journey Now." *Goodreads*, Goodreads, 2020, www.goodreads.com/quotes/427696-every-personneeds-to-take-one-day-away-a-day

[14]Salem Network. "Anapausis Meaning in Bible - New Testament Greek Lexicon - New American

Standard." *Biblestudytools.com*, 2020,
www.biblestudytools.com/lexicons/greek/nas/anapa
usis.html.

[15]Salem Network. "Rest - International Standard
Bible Encyclopedia." *Biblestudytools.com*,
2020,
www.biblestudytools.com/encyclopedias/isbe/r
est.h tml.

[16]Clark, Malissa A. "Workaholism: It's Not Just
Long
Hours on the Job." *American Psychological
Association*, American Psychological Association,
Apr. 2016,
www.apa.org/science/about/psa/2016/04/workaholis
m

[17]The Canyon. "What Is a Workaholic?" *The
Canyon*, 13 Nov. 2018,
thecanyonmalibu.com/blog/workaholic/.

Amber. "Home." *Workaholics Anonymous*, 2019,
www.workaholics-anonymous.org/10-
literature/32signposts-of-workaholism.

Drexler, Peggy. "The Dangerous Side of
Workaholism." *Forbes*, Forbes Magazine, 19
July 2013,

www.forbes.com/sites/peggydrexler/2013/07/1
9/the -dangerous-side-of-
workaholism/#458192082539.

Stillman, Jessica. "The 7 Signs of Workaholism."
Inc.com, Inc., 28 Aug. 2014,
www.inc.com/jessicastillman/the-7-signs-of-
workaholism.html.

Chapter 4 Rest for the Soul

[21]"God's grace is the healing sustenance for the
soul" Suzanne Leigh, 2020
Philippians 4:7, Psalm 91, Psalm 89:3-33, NKJV

Chapter 5 Shemita Rest

Isaiah 55:10 (NKJV), 2 Chronicles 36:21 reference
        (NKJV), Leviticus 25:2-5 (NKJV),

[22]Sendor, Noam Y. "Let the Land Rest: Lessons
        from Shmita, the Sabbatical Year." *Aytzim*,
        2020, aytzim.org/resources/articles/276.

[23]Beck, Kevin. "What Are the Six Main Elements in
        Living Organisms?" *Sciencing*, 2 Mar. 2019,
        sciencing.com/six-main-elements-living-
        organisms8155041.html.

[24]Gillespie, Claire. "Why Is Nitrogen Important for Living Things?" *Sciencing*, 2 Mar. 2019, sciencing.com/why-nitrogen-important-livingthings-4609019.html

[25]Jacobs, Rabbi Louis. "Shemitah, the Sabbatical Year, and The Jubilee Year (Yovel)." *My Jewish Learning*, 2020, www.myjewishlearning.com/article/sabbatical-yearshemitah-and-jubilee-year-yovel/.

[26]Goodreads. "A Quote by Ovid." *Goodreads*, Goodreads, 2020, www.goodreads.com/quotes/183226-take-rest-afield-that-has-rested-gives-a-beautiful.

[27]Sendor, Noam Yehuda. "Let the Land Rest: Lessons from Shemita, the Sabbatical Year (Longer Article)." *Jewcology*, 2020, jewcology.org/resources/let-the-land-rest-lessonsfrom-shemita-the-sabbatical-year-longer-article/.

[28]Odrodnick, Anna. "Why Soil Needs as Much Rest as We Do." *Fresh Harvest GA*, 21 May 2018, blog.freshharvestga.com/why-soil-needs-as-muchrest-as-we-do/.

[29]McLaughlin, Kelly. "India's Air Quality Has Improved so Much since the Country Went on Coronavirus Lockdown Citizens Can Now See

the Himalayas for the First Time in 30 Years."
Insider, Insider, 14 Apr. 2020,
www.insider.com/himalayas-seen-fromindia-
pollution-drop-coronavirus-lockdown-2020-4.

[30]Masson, Athena. "COVID-19 May Have
Temporarily
Lessened Our Carbon Footprint." *WUSF
Public
Media*, 10 Sept. 2020,
wusfnews.wusf.usf.edu/202006-15/covid-19-
may-have-temporarily-lessenedour-carbon-
footprint.

[31]Sommer, Lauren, et al. "Traffic Is Way Down
Because
Of Lockdown, But Air Pollution? Not So
Much."
NPR, NPR, 19 May 2020,
www.npr.org/sections/healthshots/2020/05/19/
854760999/traffic-is-way-downdue-to-
lockdowns-but-air-pollution-not-so-much.
[32]Mail online, Ryan Morrison For. "Air Pollution in
New York City Falls Rapidly as People Stay Home
amid Coronavirus Crisis." *Daily Mail Online*,
Associated
Newspapers, 19 Mar. 2020,
www.dailymail.co.uk/sciencetech/article81296
31/Air-pollution-New-York-City-fallsrapidly-

people-stay-home-amid-
coronaviruscrisis.html.

Chapter 6 Outcomes from Lack of Rest

Romans 10:17 (NKJV), Acts 16 (NKJV), Acts
19:10 (NKJV), Philippians 1:6 (NKJV), 1
Peter 5:7 (NKJV), Matthew 11:28-30 (NKJV).
[37]Boom, Corrie ten. "A Quote by Corrie Ten
Boom." *Goodreads*, Goodreads, 2020,
www.goodreads.com/quotes/110765-worrying-
iscarrying-tomorrow-s-load-with-today-s-
strength-carrying-two.

[38]Goodreads. "Find Quotes." *Goodreads*,
Goodreads, 2020,
www.goodreads.com/quotes/search?utf8=%E2
%9C
%93%2CPray+and+let+God+Worry+Martin+
Luthe r.

[39]Deibert, Brannon. "What Is Yoke in the Bible?
Meaning & Importance of Jesus' Teaching."
Christianity.com, Salem Web Network, 12

Feb. 2019, www.christianity.com/jesus/life-
ofjesus/teaching-and-messages/the-yoke-of-
jesusbiblical-meaning-and-importance.html.

[40]Weems, Kerri. "A Yoke for Rest?" *Faith Gateway*, 2 Nov. 2017, www.faithgateway.com/yoke-restjesus/#.XtJ8Vi5KjIU.

Chapter 7 Trust God

Psalm 95:8-10 (NKJV), Hebrews 4:1-10 (NKJV), Numbers 20:7 (NKJV), Deuteronomy 12:8-10 (NKJV), Hebrews 12:1 (NLT)

[33]Bible Hub. "Bible Hub." *Hebrews 4:10 Commentaries: For the One Who Has Entered His Rest Has Himself Also Rested from His Works, as God Did from His.*, 2004, biblehub.com/commentaries/Hebrews/4-10.htm.

[34]Merriam-Webster Incorp. "Ill Will Synonyms, Ill Will Antonyms." *Merriam-Webster*, Merriam-Webster, 2020, www.merriam-webster.com/thesaurus/ill will.

[35]Dictionary, Incorp. "Disobedience." *Dictionary.com*, Dictionary.com, 2020, www.dictionary.com/browse/disobedience.

[36]Bible Hub. "Matthew Henry's Concise Commentary." *Hebrews 4:10*, 2004,

biblehub.com/commentaries/Hebrews/4-10.htm.

Epilogue
Acts 3:19 (NKJV), 1 Corinthians 12:3 (NKJV),
Matthew 5:37 (NKJV)

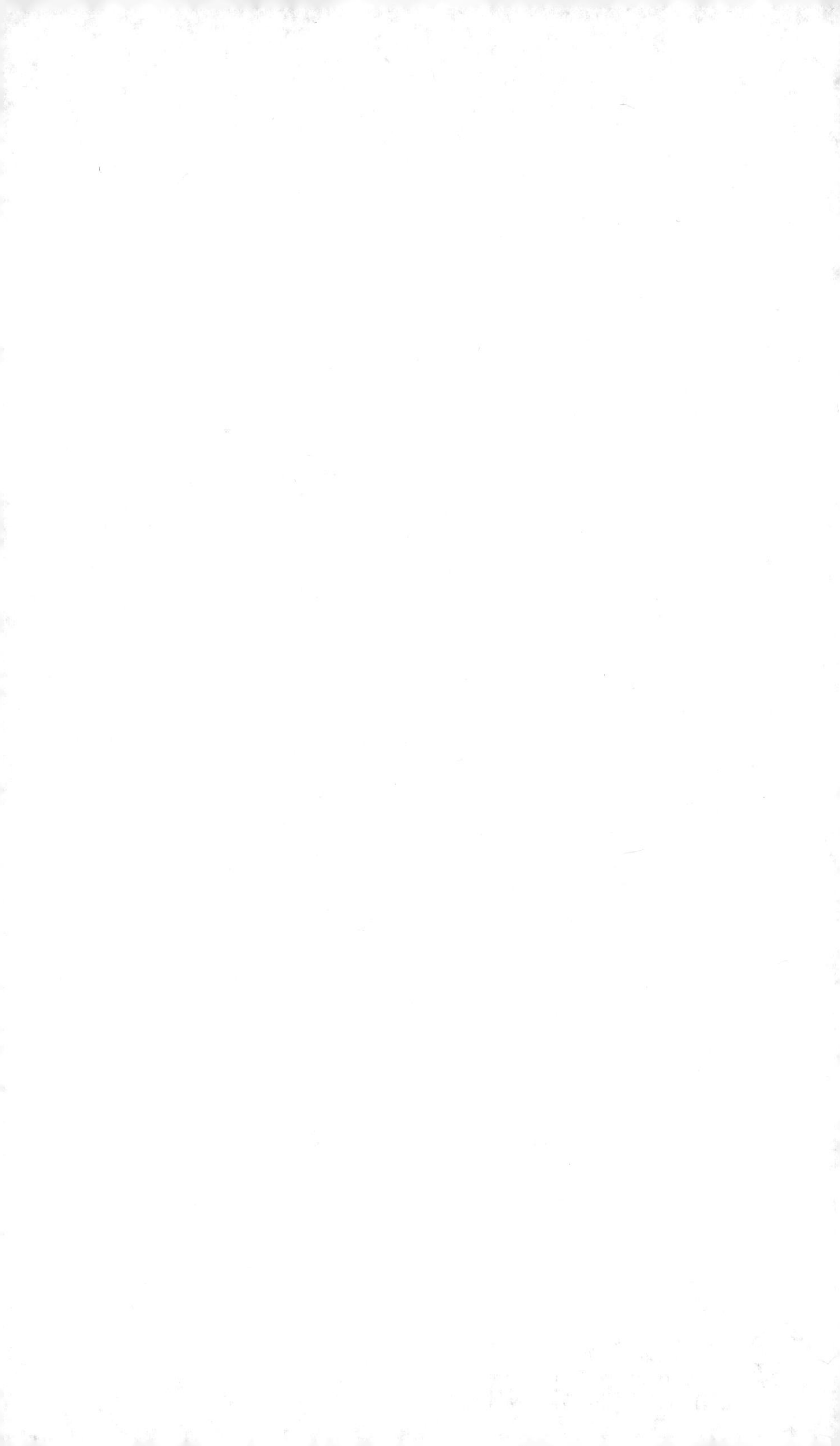